HEALTHY WEIGHT LOSS AND DIETING

Burn fat, heal your metabolism and live longer

By

Kelly P. King

Tables of contains

TAKEAWAY

CONCLUSION

INTRODUCTION

You will pick up useful knowledge.

information on effective weight loss and maintenance

a more active, healthy way of living.

Having a high body mass index may lead to several health problems.
Studies

have shown that being overweight causes hypertension and heart issues.

cancer, diabetes, sleep apnea, and other issues.

Moreover, being overweight may limit your ability to walk, run, or

take a seat in a typical chair comfortably.
There is no other way out of this situation.

is to lose the additional weight, use a healthy weight reduction strategy.

Have a strategy and adhere to it strictly.
I'll be providing you with crucial information and advice that will be useful to you.

efficiently lower your weight to more manageable levels.

Every wholesome weight-loss strategy recommended by dieticians and

Nutritionists begin by making a straightforward recommendation: eat less.

intake at the ideal level.
Nevertheless, regrettably, it is the most

a challenging task that requires significant mental effort on your part

an effort to reject the additional treats and quantities that are so

alluring.

Being cautious not to minimize is one thing to keep in mind.

you eat too rapidly, it could harm your health.

and your outcomes.

The reduced calorie intake also has other implications.

choosing a more wholesome and balanced diet. In general,

a good weight reduction diet strategy consists of fresh fruits and

combined with veggies, low-fat dairy products, nutritious grains,

consuming plenty of water—at least 8 to 10 glasses every day.

If you wish to attain your objectives, you need also to include an appropriate

an exercise program to increase lean muscle mass and burn additional calories

energy. Make it a habit to undertake some exercise for 30 minutes every day.

whether it be a quick walk around your neighborhood, a

neighborhood, an exercise at home, or a visit to your nearby fitness center

Regardless of the healthy eating program you choose, it will need to

considerable effort to lose those extra pounds, both physically and emotionally

you have put on weight over the years.
But I can promise that

The work you put in will pay off in the end.

Chapter 1

WHAT IS A DIET?

A diet is consuming a certain food selection intending to enhance your health, control your weight, or cure a sickness.

Every day, new weight loss regimens, publications, and diets are published.
Although many people need to shed a few pounds, it's crucial to stick to a diet and fitness routine you can stick with.
The strategy must support your long-term health.

Around 2 out of 3 people are overweight or obese.
The chance of developing chronic conditions including heart disease, stroke, type 2 diabetes, and several malignancies rises when you are overweight.
If you are overweight, even a few kilograms of weight loss may reduce your chance of developing health issues.

Chapter 2

HOW CAN I LOSE WEIGHT IN A HEALTHY WAY?

If your weight is outside of the recommended range, you must exercise regularly and stick to a balanced diet.
Just consume what you need to satisfy your energy demands in terms of nutrient-dense meals and beverages.

A balanced diet made up mostly of items from these 5 healthy food categories should be part of your healthy eating plan:

Vegetables and fruit of various colors

whole grains,
lean meats,
poultry fish
eggs,
tofu,
nuts,
seeds,
legumes,
beans,
milk,
yogurt,
and cheese (with mostly reduced fat)

Consuming foods with extra sugar, salt, and saturated fat should be restricted.

Together with these recommendations, you should:

Reduce your alcohol consumption.

Reduce takeout, increase regular mealtimes, and consume healthy snacks.

smaller serving sizes

have breakfast and indulge in a range of dishes

consume a lot of fiber to feel full

consume more veggies

You should engage in some kind of physical activity every day of the week as part of your healthy fitness regimen.
For adults, this involves any one of the following, alone or in combination.

12 to 5 hours of light exercise each week, such as swimming, golfing, jogging, or mowing the grass

14 to 2 12 hours a week of severe exercises, such as running, aerobics, quick cycling, soccer, or netball

Make sure your plan includes exercises that build muscle, such as push-ups, pull-ups, squats, lunges, or weights.

By using the stairs rather than the elevator or by walking or cycling instead of driving, you may include physical exercise in your day.
Keeping your sitting time to a minimum is also crucial.

Chapter 3

WHAT IS A FAD DIET?

A "fad" diet is an eating regimen that often guarantees quick weight reduction.
One thing all fad diets have in common is that they offer a short-term fix to what is, for many individuals, a chronic issue.

The media often promotes fad diets.
They often lack a scientific foundation or a substantial body of clinical data to support their assertion.
A common requirement of fad diets for weight reduction is cutting out whole food categories, which may prevent you from consuming all the nutrients your body requires.

Diets that are vegetarian or vegan should not be confused with fad diets.
These are not diets for losing weight, and vegetarians and vegans may get all the nutrients they need with careful preparation.

Chapter 4

WHAT ARE THE RISKS OF FAD DIETING?

It's crucial to understand that not all fad diets are effective, and some may pose a risk of injury.
A restricted fad diet may result in:

continuous hunger resulting in food cravings and an increased appetite slowdown of the body's metabolism (how fast you burn calories), which means you will gain weight more readily in the future

quick weight gain then rapid weight decrease

a disordered eating pattern, such as bulimia or anorexia nervosa

fewer muscles and fewer bone minerals

tiredness sleeplessness, and headaches

diarrhea or constipation lower body temperature

Lean muscle, not fat, makes up the majority of the weight you lose when following a fad diet.
The reason for this is that when you eat too little, your body breaks down muscle to receive the kilojoules it needs.
Your body can get more kilojoules from muscle than fat.

Chapter 5

HOW DO I SPOT A FAD DIET?

Australia is a prominent place for fad diets.
Fad diets often encourage rapid weight reduction without medical or dietician supervision and put a short-term emphasis on modifications to your food or exercise regimen.

Fad diets may cause you to lose weight temporarily, but they are tough to maintain.
These may result in severe health issues.
The greatest strategy for losing weight is to maintain a balanced diet over the long term and engage in regular exercise.

Chapter 6

WHAT ELSE CAN I DO TO KEEP A HEALTHY WEIGHT?

To help maintain a healthy weight, consider the following 5 steps:

Before visiting the store, have a plan for your weekly shopping.
To maintain a healthy weight, one must eat nutritious, balanced meals.
The correct foods being available at home is often the first step towards eating a balanced diet.

Substitute homemade, healthier options for meals and snacks that are rich in calories, fat, salt, and sugar.

The healthiest selections should be used when ordering takeout.
How to replace high-calorie meals with healthier options is provided by LiveLighter.

Commit to stepping up your physical activity level one more time.
Whenever feasible, adults should exercise for at least 30 minutes each day of the week at a moderate level.
Cycling or fast walking might be examples of this.
To reduce weight, you may need to exert yourself more.

For guidance, consult your physician.

the risk zones for the week.
As a result of dining out, being exhausted, or feeling worried, you may find yourself overindulging in meals rich in fat and sugar at these times.
You can restrict such foods if you organize your week.
Yet, don't be too rigorous; it's okay to indulge sometimes.

Chapter 7

DIETING FOR YOUR HEALTH AND WELL BEING

No other motivation to diet is more important than your health.

well-being and good health.
As we have covered, those of

Those of us who are overweight are more aware of the dangers and

implications that our weight may have the potential to inflict.

Yet like with smokers, the hazards aren't always obvious.

until we reach our turning point, everything is so clear-cut.
Whether

Your dietary preferences result from an addiction to certain foods, an

emotional need, or years of ingrained programming

Unless you truly alter your eating habits, nothing will change.

and your preferences.

For many individuals, dieting has evolved into a way of life in and of itself.

yo-yo-ing or quickly switching from one diet to another with little to no consistency

success and escalating despondency at an abject lack of outcomes.
The

Yet, unless you choose to accept responsibility for your mistakes and

Immediately re-join the wagon; otherwise, no diet will be successful.

successful.

An easy diet won't work, which is a sad but true fact.

make the pounds vanish suddenly while continuously depriving

You may have more of a sense of yourself and the things you love most

More likely to have an adverse than a favorable impact on your performance.

The main lesson that the majority of people need to grasp is that dieting

is not always advantageous.
What most obese individuals often do

The most important thing is to have a good lifestyle.

adjustments to their everyday schedules.
Many dismiss the idea of

even while they are options, walking the stairs or parking farther away

reasonable strategies for working in a more physical manner

your day with activities.

If they are ineffective for you, how about taking up dancing?
Seriously,

In most towns, there are beginning dancing lessons that will

dances of all ages, sizes, and fitness abilities are welcomed and invited.

You are prepared to put out the work.
Such a fantastic method to learn and becoming healthy

do something new, enjoy yourself, and avoid becoming hungry.

An additional benefit of engaging in something like a dancing class

(Take into account going ballroom dancing with your significant other)

are not inclined to eat when you are eating or are not eating

in most situations, dancing.
You are burning, which is another fantastic thing.

the energy intakes you skipped.
Try joining a group if dancing isn't your thing.

acquiring a new activity or joining a walking group. anything that motivates you

It's a good idea to stay off of your refrigerator and at your feet.

a positive development in terms of diets and weight reduction.

Remember that you cannot significantly reduce your weight.

by a strict diet.

You must make physical fitness a priority.

daily schedule to obtain those quick and aesthetically

Stunning outcomes are what you're aiming for.

People tend to give up on diets much too easily, which is another potential danger.
Some quit midway through the process or get upset that they aren't losing enough weight dramatically as soon as they had wanted, marking off yet another failure when they might have succeeded more than ever before if they had stayed with their initial diet plan a little bit longer.

The scale may be either your greatest friend or worst adversary while dieting, which is another thing you should keep in mind.
If you weigh yourself every day in the hopes of seeing the scale drop yet another pound, you are setting yourself up for failure.
If you have nightly Rocky Road or Chunky Monkey binges out of depression because you didn't drop 10 pounds overnight, you will never get the results you are looking for.

Very few diets work when it comes to weight loss.
There are, however, a lot of behavioral modifications that, when applied consistently and forcefully, are effective.

The important thing to keep in mind is that you are the one who has to put in the effort; rigorous dieting of any kind is very unlikely to help you reach the long-term outcomes you need.

Chapter 8

SIMPLY WEIGHT LOSS TIPS YOU CAN USE TO INCREASE YOUR CHANCE OF SUCCESS

You may employ a variety of strategies to effectively reduce weight and perhaps reach your weight reduction objectives.

The greatest thing you can do to lose weight is to eat healthily, as we have discussed before.

Healthy eating entails being mindful of the foods you consume, not just how much of them you consume.
When you're on a diet, you may naturally want to limit the number of items you consume, but it's more crucial to concentrate on the meals you DO eat.
For example, if you choose fruit over chips, you could have more fruit snacks with meals than you could if you just indulged in junk food.

It's not always as simple as you would assume to eat healthily.
Choose nutritious meals and become acquainted with them as one of your priorities.
You may accomplish this by browsing the Internet for information or by purchasing many cookbooks with recipes for healthy eating.

It is crucial to "spice" up your meals and make an effort to avoid eating the same meals every single day of the week to lessen the boredom that is often connected with healthy eating, particularly if you are not used to it.
I know you've heard me say this before, but it is vitally important
that you include regular exercise along if you're healthy eating plan
to achieve your weight loss goals.

Exercise is important to your success, simply because it burns off
calories.   Did you know that when you burn calories, the amount of
calories that your body absorbs decreases?

This is, essentially, what makes it possible for you to lose weight.
If you haven't been exercising regularly in the past, it is important
that you take it slow. Exercise is a great way to lose weight, but
you do not want to overdo it, especially at first.

If you don't currently have an exercise plan or program in place,
you may be wondering what you can do to get moving in the right
direction.   One of the ways that you can go about finding exercises

or workouts to do is by reading different fitness magazines. Many
fitness magazines have detailed exercises outlined in them, often
accompanied by pictures.

Another option is to find instructional workout videos that you can
do at home. You can usually find a wide variety of choices online
or at your local department store. Just remember, it is important
to start out slow or at least start with exercises that will be easy for
you to do.

Eating healthy and regular exercise are both important
components of losing weight, but there are additional tips that you
can be used to help you lose weight.

One of those tips involves finding a workout partner or a workout
buddy. This is a person who can exercise with you, whether your
exercise involves visiting a local gym or just going for a walk at a
local shopping center. Having a workout partner may help to keep
you motivated and it may help to keep exercising and losing

weight fun and exciting for you.

Another way that you can go about successfully achieving your
The weight loss goal is by "spicing," up your exercise. To help reduce
the boredom often associated with exercising you will want to
change up your exercise routine. For instance, one day you may
want to use a treadmill, the next day you may want to lift weights,
and the next day you may want to do an exercise DVD, and so
forth.

Don't be afraid to build up your lean muscle mass. Did you know
that muscles burn calories when they work; they even burn calories
when you're resting. Muscles burn calories all-day. so it only
makes that you will lose more weight by increasing your muscle
mass. The more muscles, the less fat will be left. This is attainable
starting with working out with resistance exercises.

You should also consider making an exercise and healthy eating
journals for yourself. They can be used to track your progress. If

you have a good week, like one where you completed
all of your exercises, you may want to think about rewarding
yourself. Your reward doesn't have to include food; it can be
something as simple as treating yourself to a new outfit or a night
at the movies.

Losing weight does not have to mean sacrifice and suffering. It
actually means opening up to a more full and healthy life where you
don't have to feel bad about yourself or keep yourself from doing
the things that you want to do. Losing weight might require a few
adjustments and some discomforts, but as the old saying goes,
"no pain, no gain."

Chapter 9

DECIDING WHETHER OR NOT WEIGHT LOSS SURGERY IS WORTH THE COST FOR YOU.

Did you know that if you want to shed 80 pounds or more,

You could qualify for weight-loss surgery, right?

Although it is encouraging to learn you could benefit from weight

You may be unsure about the appropriateness of weight-loss surgery.

with you.
Furthermore, you may be unsure whether losing weight would help.

Surgery is cost-effective.
If you have a query, feel free to ask.

If you want to know the solution, keep reading.

In a nutshell, the answer to the issue of whether weight reduction surgery is

worth the money has a simple response: it depends.
Despite that

That may not have been the solution you were seeking.

because that is the reality.
A lot of people find that weight reduction surgery is a good

worth it, but other people don't get anything from it.

from a weight-loss operation.
Identifying if weight loss surgery

You'll want to take certain steps that you individually feel are worth the expense of

takes several things into account.

One of the numerous things you'll want to consider is

When deciding if weight reduction surgery is worthwhile,

Your weight will cost you money.
There are a lot of weight loss

You must be at least 80 pounds overweight to have surgery.

undertake a weight-loss operation.
In light of this, you may be able to

finding a surgeon who will make an exception is possible, but it doesn't mean

not imply that you should choose surgery.
If it's possible

You may reduce your weight by yourself, through exercise, and

You could discover that eating healthily is considerably more economical to accomplish.

You should also consider other factors, such as your health.

taking into account while deciding if weight reduction surgery

suitable for you.
The term "weight loss surgery" is often used.

health-saving operation.
Those that are very fat place

their health is in jeopardy, and they can pass away too soon.
When you are

If you are really fat, your doctor could advise losing weight.

surgery.

If so, weight reduction surgery is more than worthwhile.

the expenses, since your health and safety cannot be placed a price on.

feeling good.

Another aspect to consider is your capacity to develop and stick to objectives.

When deciding if weight reduction surgery is cost-effective, take into account
to you.
You might lose weight quickly with weight loss surgery,

But, weight loss will not be aided by the procedure alone.
With a smaller

The majority of weight-loss procedures use a stomach pouch,

You must restrict how much food you consume.
Until you do so,

You can put your health at risk and put on weight again.

still more.
If you don't believe you can adhere to all of the

While receiving instructions after your weight reduction surgery, it

may not be your best choice.

These are just a handful of the many elements that must be

before determining whether weight reduction surgery is the best option for you.

or whether the price is justified.
Also, I want you to be aware that not all

People can have weight reduction surgery, and I am one of them.

not a doctor or other medical expert.
I do not wholeheartedly support

any kind of weight-loss surgery.
This article was solely intended to

assist you in weighing your alternatives.

If you believe that having weight reduction surgery might benefit your

You must take the time to speak with your attorney about the problem.

research and consult a doctor.

Chapter 10

HOW TO USE THE INTERNET DEVELOP YOUR WEIGHT LOSS PLAN

It's possible to create your own in a variety of methods.

weight loss program.
You may enroll in a weight-loss program already in place,

You could discover the expense of programs like Weight Watchers or Nutrisystem

spending a little bit more than you're willing to accomplish so, particularly if

Your spending is limited.
So, a lot of people decide to grow their

personal diet programs.

Creating a self-care weight reduction strategy for the first time might be challenging.

Maybe you are unsure about the best course of action.
Why is

The benefit of creating a personal weight reduction strategy is that you

be liberated.
However, you'll still want to check to make sure

you can take advantage of and profit from your weight-loss strategy.

that while using, you might reduce your weight. Because of this, you might

If you want to grow, you may want to consider using the Internet.

a weight-loss regimen or strategy that is uniquely your own.

While creating your weight-loss strategy, there are many things to consider.

The Internet may benefit you in many different ways.

assistance.
First of all, a crucial component of any weight reduction

The program includes eating well.
Eating is a common activity.

It's a little strange to talk about being healthy, just because

They lack knowledge on what to prepare or how to cook it.

Online, you may discover a variety of websites, many of which are

providing access to healthful foods, which are free to use, and

recipes.
Some of these recipes include pictures, so you can

ought should be able to determine if the questioned food is safe immediately.

is a substance you would consume.

Exercise is a different component of weight loss to some.

Those who want to reduce weight might do it by just going for a stroll.

Others must engage in more vigorous activity to lose weight.

activities.
If you fit that description, there is a

Several websites include instructions for activities that you should be able to do.

There are a ton of websites dedicated to fitness that you'll probably discover.

Having specific images or videos that demonstrate each stage of the process in detail,the exercise in question.

Ordering weight reduction products from the Internet is another option.

fitness gear, weight loss books, or videos.
Good things

a suggestion on how to use the Internet to locate workout tools

You may implement this strategy into your at-home weight reduction regimen.

You may read product reviews online in addition to making purchases.

Reviewing products is a fantastic approach to finding out whether a workout tool is worth buying.

That interests you is a good investment.

As soon as you have identified a handful of activities that you

You should also prepare a couple of nutritious meals.

Make yourself a list or keep a notebook; it's a smart idea.

to your workout regimen like a timetable.
Using this as an example

Describe the exercise you want to do each Monday.

your preferences for the meals you want to consume on that day.
To have a

a weekly schedule for weight reduction with specific goals for each day

the likelihood that you will stick to your strategy will be increased.

The Internet, as you can see, is a useful resource to have when you are

getting ready to design your diet.
Do not forget that

Everyone can create their at-home diet plan.

heed it, then.
If you discover that it is tough for you to remain

Consider attending a local weight reduction program to keep your progress on track.

locate at least one local weight loss program, an online weight reduction program, or

a reliable friend who can keep you on course.

Chapter 11

USING COLON CLEANSES TO HELP YOU LOSE WEIGHT

Diet pills are frequently what most of us consider when looking for weight loss products.

the first idea that occurs to you.
While diet medications could be helpful to

Diet pills are used by some individuals to assist them to reach their weight reduction objectives.

not the only accessible weight-loss product.
This afternoon, we'll

discuss weight loss programs and colon cleansing.

loss cleanses and perhaps will enable you to determine whether or not may support weight loss.

There are many options available for utilizing colon cleanses to reduce weight.

Many people, probably including you, are curious about how the whole

The method works.
Before learning about how colon cleansing may

it's vital to keep in mind that there may not be any effective methods to be different.
Several colon-cleansing products promote this.

They are made to assist you in losing weight.
As I already said

Other names for various kinds of colon cleanses include

Cleanses for losing weight.
There are colon cleanses to help with this.

that declare they cannot promise to help you lose weight,even if some of them may.

You must carefully adhere to the directions provided while utilizing a colon cleanse.

every instruction that was provided to you.
As an example, there are several

Using a colon cleanse that calls for a one- to two-day fast

both days.
These cleanses for the colon often come in liquid form.

Then there are colon cleanses that come in tablet form.

In many cases

recommend sticking to particular foods and beverages alone, such as clear liquids produce, and grains.

If you purchase a colon cleanse that requires you to limit your food and

It is a good idea to follow the directions exactly if you want it to perform successfully.

following the recommended diet to the letter.
The dietary limitation is

What enables you to reduce weight, as well as enables the colon cleanse to function well.

You are effectively detoxing when you do a colon cleanse,

the body.
Toxins will be expelled from the body by the colon cleanse.

sometimes even your intestines, including your colon.
Not only that, but

good for promoting well-being, but it may also aid in weight loss

weight.
According to some reports, the typical human has somewhere

from four to eight pounds of accumulated garbage. When

That additional waste will be eliminated from your body with a colon cleanse.

This is why a lot of people are successful in losing weight by by use of a colon cleanse.

If you can employ a quick colon cleansing, such as one

You might see a significant weight decrease in three to seven days.
Ones that

Some people who want to reduce weight rapidly utilize colon cleanses

before a major occasion, such as a wedding or trip. when you

may be able to lose weight quickly with a colon cleanse, however

You must use prudence as you go forward.
If you don't alter

If you change the way you eat or include exercise in your routine, you

you might regain some of your weight in as little as a few weeks or months.

Usually, if you were instructed to limit your diet while

by use of a colon cleanse.
While you are not required to keep up with your

Reduce your consumption of junk food if you follow a limited diet.

and begin a daily or at the very least weekly fitness regimen.

Therefore it is quite likely that a colon cleanse can help you lose weight

you may be interested in trying one to detoxify.
When you search

You may be able to find them available for purchase as a colon cleanse for

sale in a nearby department store, health food store, or vitamin store

offline and online.

You may want to think again before investing in a colon cleanse.

can look for product reviews online or get in touch with a healthcare

professional.
If you purchase a colon, doing so will assist to guarantee that

Ensure that your money is being wisely used.

Chapter 12

DECIDING WHETHER OR NOT YOU SHOULD USE WEIGHT LOSS PILLS YOUR DIET PLAN.

If you've been struggling to lose weight, there's a good possibility that you've thought about using weight loss (diet) tablets at least once.
Today, we'll strive to assist you in determining if you need to.
Please bear in mind that I am not a medical expert.

I also don't wholeheartedly support the usage of any kind of medicine or dietary supplement.

You can only use the information in this issue to make wise decisions.

Having said that, there are several different questions that you will want to ask yourself to determine whether or not weight loss pills are the best choice for you.
Hopefully, these questions will enable you to decide whether using diet pills is the best course of action for you.

One of the numerous questions you should ask yourself is if you want to stop losing weight.
Exercise and a good diet are often required for "natural" weight loss.

Have you been working out?

While I may sound like a harp, you must move if you don't want to lose.
Exercise doesn't need to be painful.
Simple things like going for a quick stroll or dancing around the house for 30 minutes might count as exercise.

Also, have you been eating well?

Cutting down significantly on sweets and processed food is part of eating healthfully.
then substitute lots of fruits and vegetables in their place!

If you haven't already done so, I strongly advise that you first attempt natural weight loss methods before turning to any kind of medication.

While many factors might contribute to weight gain, overeating is one of the most frequent causes.
So, you must ask yourself why you overeat.
Do you eat only out of boredom or is it necessary for your body?

recognize your hunger?

You must respond to this crucial question since many,

Your appetite will be reduced with weight reduction tablets.
Although this

may assist you in lowering the quantity of food you consume and the

Only if you believe that counting calories benefits you.

even after you have eaten, your body is constantly signaling to you that you eaten a whole meal.

Whether you eat solely out of boredom or for another reason,

then there is a strong possibility that you will still have an underlying explanation.

Even if you are using an appetite suppressor, keep eating.

Are you aware of another crucial factor that you should take into account?

prepared to cope with the negative impacts of weight loss pills.

The chemicals in various diet pills vary, so their adverse effects

impact varies.

The majority of prescription diet adverse effects

headache, irritation, muscular tension, and dizziness are side effects of medications.

nausea, jitters, and anxiety.
other mild side effects

include indigestion, dry mouth, and sleeplessness due

These medications' ingredients also affect how a person sleeps.

The neurological system is often stimulated by appetite suppressants, which

may increase heart rate and blood pressure.
This ups the chance of

cardiac arrest and heart attacks, particularly in those who

already experience irregular heartbeat, high blood pressure, or

coronary disease.

Regarding fat-blocking medications like orlistat that eliminate extra fat via

they may cause unpleasant cramps, gas, and bloating in the intestines.

diarrhea.
Since these medicines also decrease the body's ability to absorb

Those who consume them are adequate sources of vital vitamins and minerals.

suggested taking a daily dosage of multivitamins.

Although being "all-natural," herbal diet medications might have

Depending on their severity, possible negative effects

ingredients.
But remember that "Herbal" doesn't always

also because they are regarded as food, meaning "safe."

industry, which the FDA regulates differently, there is no

assurance that they will fulfill the promises made by their producers.

On the surface, diet pills may seem to be the perfect remedy for

shedding pounds.
There is one additional consideration you should make, however.

Keep in mind that when you consume fewer calories, your metabolism slows.

also slows.
Your metabolism slows down, causing you to gain weight.

You slow down as well.

This is why it's typical for individuals to only lose a particular amount of weight.

weight when using just diet tablets.
The remedy, of

of course, is to implement little lifestyle adjustments, such as frequent

Exercise, a good diet, and regular checks may considerably

amplify your success.

Just a friendly reminder that you must follow the correct procedures

Do your homework before buying any weight-loss products.
Do not forget that

While not all weight loss supplements are made similarly, there are

various outcomes.
Dietary supplement risks should always be considered

weighed before making a choice.

Chapter 13

DEVELOPING AN EFFECTIVE   WEEKLY EXERCISE

The purpose of creating a weekly schedule is to enable you to:

to create both a regular strategy for weight reduction and

when it comes to exercise, a healthy endurance.

Your attention must be focused on program planning and implementation.

Thus you'll need to be ready mentally and emotionally.

As I've said previously, I strongly suggest that you go

Before beginning any workout, see your doctor for a checkup.

While creating your own, one crucial thing to keep in mind

Stretching should be included in your workout routine.

both before and after your workout session.
strengthening your muscles

To prevent any injuries or stiffness, it's necessary to stretch the body.

You should also start gently.
All actions should be taken quickly.

moderation.
Choose the degree of training and activity that is right for you.

You should have just enough space to be cozy without having too much.

It's handy that it won't provide a significant issue.

I'll use the first week of your life as an example.

maybe a part of the program.

On the first day of the program, participants take a lengthy, steady walk in a

a little more than 20 minutes.
Have a decent nap after the stroll.

On the first day, this hardly consumes any of your time.
With less

You have already begun the process of losing weight in less than an hour.

a program that may be advantageous to you.

Focusing on an upper body exercise by the second day is a smart idea.

This keeps your strength up so you can endure the whole

The weekly schedule.

On the third day, you should jog or walk quickly for 10 minutes.
For

novice, lower body exercise is best performed in the evening.

On the fourth day, a nice stretch and some relaxation are required.

Beginning the fifth day is a decent ten-minute stroll. Work out the

Squats, lunges, or modest weightlifting with the lower body should come next.

with an additional ten-minute walk.

On the sixth day, engage in a low-impact workout, such as:

If feasible, go swimming or even just strolling.

Never be scared to try something new to prevent becoming bored.
one last

Weekdays are ideal for going for a light-body stroll.

workout.

This is just one example of a good training regimen that you

is employable.
To fit your schedule, you may need to modify this strategy, however

The most crucial thing to keep in mind is developing and adhering to a

Your ability to attain will be greatly aided by a good workout regimen.

your aims for losing weight.

Chapter 14

VARIOUS TYPES OF WEIGHT LOSS SUPPLEMENTS.

According to studies, individuals often spend hundreds or even

Every year, hundreds of dollars are spent in the

hoping to increase their metabolism.
The industry of fitness is

rising, however despite this many individuals still struggle to lose weight

of all the diet and fitness tools at their disposal.

Did you realize that more than 60% of people in America are

are fat, with 30% of the population being overweight?
In the

An estimated 50 million individuals in the US alone are attempting to

Sadly, just 5% of those who attempt to reduce weight are successful.

Several weight loss products make false promises about their

The details on the supplements available today are

hazy at best.
Manufacturers of dietary supplements depend on the

due to the reality that most individuals merely want a fast cure, they

jumping from one product to another to

the outcomes they want.

Nowadays, there are a huge number of weight reduction products available.

incorporating the
Diet Patch was discontinued by the FDA in the 1990s.

since they are useless.
Magnetic diet pills are said to drain fat away, but they don't.

Guar gum obstructs the inside of the body.

Electrical Muscle Stimulators: No impact has been shown.

- Appetite-Suppressing Glasses - They state that the

appetite is reduced by a projected picture on the retina.

Weight loss earrings that restrict appetite thanks to acupuncture

Then there are diet beverages that may be used in place of meals.

The disadvantage to this is that if you stop drinking, you'll

within a short time, restore the weight loss.
Here are a few You may know:

Herbalife Nutritional Program: Dieters may use it as two meals.

may use shakes and adhere to artificial dieting techniques.

Nestlé's Sweet Success advises taking it three times daily.

a day and does not encourage healthy eating practices.

Extremely Slim Fast: This program calls for consistent exercise but does not

not promote healthy eating.

We now have purported natural cures.
often referred to as

formulas for natural weight reduction.
They are yet another industry inside

Unproven diet supplements dominate the market.

long-term.
Here are a few examples:

Chromium Supplements: These items promise to reduce blood

cholesterol, sugar, and body fat, although they sometimes induce
anemia

and even forgetfulness.
Studies demonstrate little to none

a positive outcome at all.

Items made from green tea extract are powerful antioxidants.

that support weight loss and reduce cholesterol and triglycerides

Nonetheless, the presence of caffeine may lead to sleeplessness and restlessness.

Spirulina includes important nutrients that may be found in algae tablets.

be a suitable complement to meals when used as a part of a diverse

However, they may come at a high price.

- St. John's Wort Supplement - Promises to reduce

Increasing your hunger might help you lose weight, but it can also

stomach pain, exhaustion, insomnia, and

elicit allergic responses.

According to Glucomannan Products, two capsules before

Food absorption reduces with each meal.
The term "food thickeners"

but not yet shown to be secure or efficient. Losing weight will only take place

if a healthy diet is followed.

Moreover, some manufacturers may advertise their goods as

include EGCG, a substance present in green tea. such that

component asserts to increase metabolism and some

Studies indicate that it can marginally increase the risk of burning.

calories and some research indicate that a significant portion of weight reduction

accomplished was not due to muscle loss but rather genuine fat reduction.

I'd say that green tea shouldn't be consumed.

considered a stand-alone weight-loss treatment, although it could

via increasing fat oxidation, in the decrease of fat tissue

and the thermogenesis that it encourages.

Alone, this raises the

muscular tissue-to-fat ratio, which encourages a greater metabolic rate

increase the rate of fat burning.

Several more advantages are also being revealed.

EGCG (green tea), which has advantages for blood sugar,

cholesterol's antioxidant effects, foul breath, and other consequences.

In the end, even if you want to use over-the-counter medications

even with weight-loss tablets, you'll need to consume fewer calories.

then you expend to lose weight.
Please use caution whenever

selecting any dietary supplements for weight reduction.
conduct research, and

gather as much data as you can to enable you to make an

a wise and healthy decision.

Chapter 15

DECIDING WHETHER OR NOT HYPNOSIS IS AN EFFECTIVE WEIGHT-LOSS TREATMENT.

managing your weight and preventing unneeded weight gain

An essential component of avoiding numerous problems, particularly as you age

health issues associated with obesity.

Are you aware that being 20 pounds or more above your optimum

Being overweight may increase your chances of possibly fatal

diseases include diabetes, hypertension, and coronary

obstructive sleep apnea, endometrial cancer, heart disease, and ovarian cancer.

Being overweight and leading a sedentary lifestyle puts you at risk for

increased chance of developing cardiovascular disease and other illnesses.

If you already suffer from a health issue like high cholesterol,

Being overweight increases your chances of other problems.

complications.

The good news is that weight reduction of any size may

your health will drastically improve.
10% of your body weight may be lost

lower high blood pressure, triglycerides, and cholesterol

levels of blood sugar.

There are several techniques available now that may assist and contribute.

Many successfully shed pounds.
One of the widely used methods in

Hypnosis is a method for weight loss.

Yet, there are a lot of misunderstandings about the

the use of hypnosis in weight loss.
Furthermore, since it doesn't

entail medication of any type and surgery, many

Many often believe that hypnosis makes it easier to lose weight.

be a reasonably secure method for losing weight.

If you're thinking about using hypnosis to lose weight, it's important to

It's crucial to learn as much as you can about its impacts.
Now, let's

simply discuss a few statistics that will provide you with some insight.

Hypnosis may be dangerous if performed incorrectly by someone who is not skilled.

Many individuals tend to believe that hypnosis won't be dangerous to

Notwithstanding their health, it is crucial to understand that the individual who will

that the person doing the surgery is knowledgeable and competent enough

things to think about before doing the operation.

An individual cannot lose weight via hypnosis alone.

The majority of medical professionals believe that hypnosis should only be used as

the method of losing weight.
It should never serve as the only method.

Loss of weight process.

Also, bear in mind that just receiving one session of

The effects of hypnosis on a person's weight are negligible.

To lose weight, hypnosis combined with psychotherapy

greater than hypnosis by itself.
This is due to hypnosis being a

just a very relaxed state of mind that one may yet be in

the ability to govern one's own body.

One method of accessing a person's subliminal state is hypnosis.

person.

During the "hypnotic stage," a person's body is

As a result of its intensified state, it is more susceptible to suggestibility. a level of attention.

But this does not necessarily imply that one can achieve hypnosis.

You can completely "reprogram" someone's mind to stop thinking.

eating unhealthy food.

In general, hypnosis is a very comfortable and natural mental state that
usually happens twice daily for most people.
It is an idyllic distance away.

an emotion that sometimes occurs just before we drop off to

Throughout the night or right before waking up in the morning, sleep is recommended.

The hypnotic condition exposes the subconscious mind's seat of

our routines to recommendations.
These recommendations strengthen our strength.

replace our negative habits with good ones.

For many people, hypnosis is a great technique for breaking undesirable behaviors.

and producing quality ones.
Hypnosis may deliver potently

subconscious cues to consume wholesome, healthful meals.

Asking the right questions is crucial with any weight-loss technique.

suggest healthy eating and exercise to your doctor.

A healthy mind is a healthy body, as the saying goes.

Chapter 16

DECIDING WHETHER OR NOT JOINING A PAID WEIGHT LOSS PROGRAM IS FOR YOU.

You will discover that you have a choice when it comes to weight reduction programs.

There are several alternatives.
Two of your most typical choices

Investing in or creating your weight reduction regimen should be considered.

We've spoken about this previously.

If you're trying to lose weight "seriously" for the first time, you

maybe unsure whether you should grow your weight

losing strategy or investing in one.
One of the most effective techniques to decide whether

The best weight-loss strategy is to consider the advantages and disadvantages.

of every.
We're going to discuss some of the benefits and

negative aspects of purchasing one.

When it comes to funding a program to lose weight, such as;

You'll discover that using Weight Watchers, Nutrisystem, or Jenny Craig

Usually, you may do this offline or online.
If you decide to take part

In a neighborhood weight reduction program, you'll probably meet in a central location.

location.
You just get together every week or two a lot of the time.

If you decide to enroll in an online program for weight reduction, you will

likely to have online conferences or conversations with instructors or other

participants in a weight reduction program, either on a message board or

by way of emails.
You need to have access to wholesome recipes as well.

and simple workouts.

One of the several benefits of investing in a weight reduction program

With a weight reduction regimen, you often get expert advice plan.

The people or coaches in charge of running often

These initiatives are trained in or have personal experience with losing weight.

This often avoids trial and error, as many others have previously done.

discovered what works and what does not.

Indeed, the only drawback to paying to join a weight reduction program

You must pay to participate in the program.
In light of that, it ought to

You may select from a variety of reasonably priced programs with relative ease.

that, both locally and online, will satisfy your demands.

If you can't afford to pay for a program or don't want to,

You can always create your strategy.
like we have

As was previously said, there are many benefits to producing

your scheme.
One benefit is that you can personalize.

your personalized program.

For instance, if you have a nut or milk allergy, you may work your

a sponsored weight loss program may not include an allergy in your strategy, while

Make the process simple.
Also, you may alter your routines to

easier to work into your schedule.

Another of the numerous benefits of creating your own

The diet is enjoyable to follow.
There are many

You may get information on weight loss on websites and periodicals.

sources and utilize them to make your unique strategy.
You could

even learn that coming up with your diet would help you more

enthused about the procedure and increase your likelihood of seeing the

Make a thorough strategy.

Of course, the choice is entirely yours.
a majority

The most crucial thing to keep in mind is to act, whether it be

either designing your weight reduction program or joining a commercial one.

Chapter 17

THE DANGERS ASSOCIATED WITH RAPID WEIGHT LOSS.

Quick weight reduction is another name for rapid weight loss.

or rapid weight reduction entails dropping a significant quantity of weight.

in a brief period, often between two and seven days.

Many thousands of people, alone in the United States, each year suffer from

Individuals are motivated to lose weight quickly. Numerous them

wishing to reduce weight before a significant occasion, such as an impending

wedding or vacation.
Although fast weight loss is achievable,

It's critical to use prudence.

The very fact that it is possible to reduce weight rapidly in a

That doesn't always imply it's healthy for you if it's just temporary.

Rapid weight reduction has risks attached to it.

For example, it is frequent to hear about people who have

To reduce weight, I decided to fast.
Do you realize that

Even for a little time, going without meals may be

risky to your health.
A better option would be to reduce

back on the food you do consume, or to focus on consuming a

good eating habits and avoiding junk food.

Healthy eating is just one aspect of weight reduction; another is exercise.

exercise.
Sure, I am aware that I have already said this, but sadly, many

Many are unaware that to lose weight, you must exercise.

weight.

While exercise is a crucial part of weight loss, it is

It's crucial to not push yourself too hard, particularly if you haven't had a

routine fitness program.
three hours spent on the treadmill,

instead of 30 minutes, which might aid in lowering your calorie consumption, however

Also, it can put you in the hospital.

Rapid weight loss is also often accompanied by another issue, which is

the use of drugs or other weight-loss supplements.
a good

The good news is that many of these items do function, and some even

safe, but it's possible you won't know what you're receiving.
When you are

interested in utilizing a weight-loss supplement or product, such as a

You must follow the cleanse to assist you in losing weight.

adequate quantity of research beforehand.
This study might entail

examining product reviews to determine the effectiveness of the purchase, or

conversing with a medical expert.

As you can see, it's crucial to use care while attempting to lose weight quickly.
Despite unforeseen circumstances or

appearances do occur, but most people get at least a month's notice.

before attending a significant event, such as a wedding or

even a getaway.
As soon as you are aware of your impending

If that happens, it is suggested that you begin your weight-loss efforts at that time.

I'm eager to accomplish it.
Losing weight quickly might be risky;

As a result, you need to avoid depending on it.

Chapter 18

EATING MINDFULLY

Those who practice mindful eating are conscious of when, where, and how they eat.
Those that engage in this behavior may be able to maintain a healthy weight while still enjoying their cuisine.
Reliable Source.

Due to their hectic schedules, the majority of individuals often eat rapidly while driving, working at their desks, or watching TV.
As a consequence, many individuals consume with little awareness of what they are doing.

The following are methods for mindful eating:

As you sit down to eat, ideally at a table, pay attention to the food and take pleasure at the moment.

Distraction-free dining: Don't use your phone, laptop, or TV while you're eating.

Eat it slowly so you have time to chew it and enjoy it.

This method aids in weight reduction because it allows the brain time to register feelings of fullness, which may help people avoid overeating.

Make thoughtful food selections: Choose meals and snacks that are high in nutritious nutrients that will keep you satisfied for hours rather than minutes.

Chapter 19

GETTING A GOOD NIGHT'S SLEEP

Much research has shown that having less than 5 to 6 hours of sleep per night is linked to a higher prevalence of obesityTrusted Source.
This is due to several factors.

Insufficient or poor-quality sleep may impede metabolism, the body's process of converting calories into energy. This is supported by research.
Unused energy may be stored as fat by the body when metabolism is less efficient.
Moreover, insufficient sleep may lead to a rise in the hormones cortisol and insulin, both of which promote the accumulation of fat.

The regulation of the hormones leptin and ghrelin, which govern hunger, is also influenced by how much sleep a person gets.
The brain receives fullness cues from leptin.

Chapter 20

MANAGING YOUR STRESS LEVELS

As part of the body's fight-or-flight reaction, stress causes the production of chemicals like adrenaline and cortisol, which at first suppress hunger.

Yet, chronic stress may cause cortisol to stay in the system for a longer period, increasing hunger and perhaps causing individuals to eat more.

Cortisol alerts the body that it needs to replace its nutritional reserves with its preferred fuel, carbohydrates.

After then, insulin delivers the blood's sugar from carbs to the muscles and brain.
The body will retain this sugar as fat if it is not used during a person's fight or flight response.

The body mass index (BMI) of children and adolescents who are overweight or obese was significantly reduced as a consequence of adopting an 8-week stress-management intervention program, according to research.

Among the techniques for reducing stress are:

Breathing exercises and relaxation methods such as yoga, meditation, or tai chi

spending time in the fresh air, such as walking or
gardening

FIND YOUR INNER MOTIVATION

Others cannot force you to lose weight.
To make yourself happy, you must make dietary and activity adjustments.
What will give you the intense motivation to follow through with your weight-loss plan?

Create a list of your priorities to keep you motivated and concentrated, whether it's a future vacation or improved general health.
Next, figure out a technique to guarantee that you can use your motivating elements when faced with temptation.
You could wish to leave a motivational message for yourself on the refrigerator or pantry door, for example.

While you must be accountable for your actions to lose weight, having the appropriate type of support may be helpful.
Choose your supporters carefully; they should boost your confidence and not cause you any humiliation or sabotage.

Find friends who will ideally listen to your worries and emotions, spend time working out with you or

preparing nutritious meals, and value living a better lifestyle as much as you do.
Accountability from your support group is another benefit that may help you stay committed to your weight-loss objectives.

If you want to keep your weight-loss ambitions a secret, hold yourself responsible by regularly checking your weight, keeping a log of your food and exercise progress, or utilizing digital tools to monitor your progress.

TAKEAWAY

It's crucial to keep in mind that there are no magic solutions for losing weight.

Eating a balanced, healthy diet is the greatest method to control weight.

Ten servings of fruit and vegetables, healthy grains, and lean protein should all be included.
Also, it is recommended to exercise daily for at least 30 minutes.

CONCLUSION

It has always been important to us to feel and look beautiful.

We become more self-aware as we get older and become adults.

Several dieting techniques are tried by us.

Infrequently, we adhere to trends and fads.

For the sake of obtaining the ideal figure, we compete with our friends, coworkers, and even ourselves.

Everything is shown on television, we hear about how individuals lose weight in the news, and we come across these weight-loss goods.

For the most part, they are ineffective.

Even if everyone still suffers from diets, this article has already provided the fundamental guidelines for effective weight loss.

Although some individuals may already be working on it, for others who are still debating whether to give it a go, have faith that your efforts will be rewarded with better outcomes.

In addition to eating healthy foods, it is advised that you also take pleasure in them.

While it is simpler to lose weight, we also highlight the importance of developing the habit of enjoying excellent meals.

When weight reduction is sustained without affecting general health, weight control measures may be effective.

When you complete a weight loss program successfully, you encourage long-lasting lifestyle modifications.

Maintaining the proper weight has both physical and psychological advantages, provided it is done correctly.
Yet tailoring a weight loss program to a person's requirements and way of life is more advantageous.

You're more likely to achieve your ideal weight when you include the proper elements of a weight-loss diet, such as sleep and exercise.
We understand that maintaining a healthy weight also shields us from several ailments.
Moreover, we operate well under pressure every day.
When we do our tasks well, we succeed.

The importance of looking nice is unquestionable for all of us.
We achieve our ideal level of health, which gives you the glow you deserve, by consuming the right nourishment and knowing how the body functions.
Sometimes we just fail to see the techniques that allow the worst parts of ourselves to win.
We don't know how to become healthy and look attractive, thus we fail to figure it out.
Being aware of our weight and look is thus not at all harmful.
The way we spend our lives and develop into useful beings is reflected in it.
You have more functioning when you are healthy.

www.ingramcontent.com/pod-product-compliance
Lightning Source LLC
Chambersburg PA
CBHW061603250726
48657CB00017B/1750